STOP DIETING NOW!

---

25 Reasons to Stop, 25 Ways to Heal

---

by Golda Poretsky, H.H.C.

Stop Dieting Now!
25 Reasons To Stop, 25 Ways To Heal

ISBN: 978-0-578-05791-0

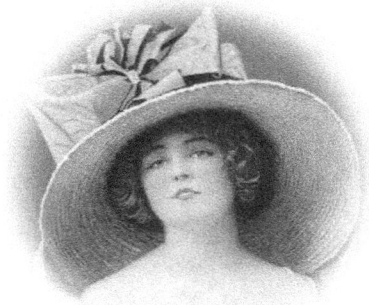

To the fat girls of the future,
may you never need a book like this!

Praise for the
Body Love Wellness Blog

"Golda is a wonderful spokesperson for Health At Every Size. Her writing is always a great combination of impassioned persuasion and practical advice and inspiration."
—**Linda Bacon, PhD**, nutrition researcher/professor and author of *Health At Every Size: The Surprising Truth About Your Weight*

"I love Golda Poretsky's Body Love Wellness Blog, one of the best out there teaching people to accept themselves and be happier and healthier at any size. If we all took her advice, we'd stop measuring our worth in pounds and inches, and make peace with the bodies we actually have, not a fictitious body that our fatphobic society wants to convince us we should want. We'd be happier, healthier, and have a lot more fun in our lives!"
—**Bill Fabrey**, NAAFA founder, 1969, Council on Size & Weight Discrimination, Membership Chair, Association for Size Diversity and Health

"Golda Poretsky is one of the most creative, intuitive, and sensitive counselors there is. Her ability to connect with people and communicate to them the skills they need to learn to start loving themselves—mind, body and all—is effective, honed and nothing short of awe-inspiring. I've personally been changed by Golda's presence in my life, as have the myriad people who read Golda's expert advice at More of Me to Love every single day."
—**Jay Solomon**, creator of *More of Me to Love*

"Body Love Wellness injects a much needed antidote of healthy self-esteem and body image into an ever increasingly disordered culture. Blogger Golda Poretsky combines both her professional expertise and lived experiences to show readers that one's self worth can't be measured by the numbers on a scale. Smart, sassy and inspirational, Body Love Wellness helps readers to change the world, not their bodies."
—**Rachel Richardson**, The F-Word Blog (www.the-f-word.org)

Acknowledgements

I have immense gratitude for my clients, who continually inspire me with their questions and successes. Thank you also to all of you blog commenters, Facebook fans and Twitter followers who continually engage me in the conversation of what it means to heal from dieting.

I want to thank the sister goddesses of Mama Gena's School of Womanly Arts, for pushing me to create the life I desire. I would also like to thank the members of NAAFA and ASDAH who continue to fight to end discrimination against fat people and encourage an understanding of size diversity and health at every size. Thank you to Marilyn Wann for encouraging me to write a book that people can read in the bathroom.

I'd like to thank my family for believing in me even when they think I'm crazy. And finally, I'd like to thank my boyfriend Jeff for believing in me even when I think I'm crazy.

And one more... a very special thanks to P.J. DeGenaro, writer and artist extraordinaire, for her invaluable help in editing, formatting and designing this book!

CONTENTS

INTRODUCTION

We are all living under the weight of a dangerous lie.

Everything—from billboards to television to bottled water labels—tells us that dieting is good, that it works, and that striving to be thin is healthy.

This lie is dangerous because it creates so much pain. From the physical pain of starving, binging and over-exercising, to the mental pain of feeling out of control around food, to the emotional pain of body hatred and weight obsession, diets (no matter what they're called) create the opposite of health of health and happiness.

By reading this book, you are waking up from the lie. I promise you that the truth is better than you expect. All I ask is that you keep an open mind and heart as you turn the pages of this book.

Is This Book For You?

If you're picking up this book and reading it, then you're in one of three places in your life right now. You've:

- gotten sick of dieting and want some validation for your desire to quit dieting for good (a "No Diet Desirer");

- stopped dieting and are looking for reinforcement in your decision (a "Non–Dieter"); or

- are still in the honeymoon phase of your current diet, think you've found what works for you, and figure that the writer of this book must be nuts (a "Dieter").

Whether you're a Dieter, a Non-Dieter or a No Diet Desirer, this book is, in fact, for you.

No Diet Desirers, if this book doesn't push you out of that Weight Watchers meeting and start you on your journey to intuitive eating, I don't know what will. Use this book to support your intuitive sense that dieting is not for you. Show it to friends, colleagues, and family. Have it at the ready whenever someone wants you to try yet another diet.

Non-Dieters, kudos to you for finding your way out of the dieting wilderness and into reality! Use this book to steel your resolve and support the decision you've already made. Wave it like garlic in the faces of dieting vampires.

Dieters, I have only one request. Keep reading this book. I know you're loving your diet right now. But trust me, unless you're in the statistically tiny group of people for whom dieting actually works, you will likely find yourself in one of the above categories soon enough. So stay engaged with this book and be willing to consider reasons why maybe—just maybe—your love affair with your diet is bound for a tragic divorce.

How To Use This Book

When I first wrote this book, I focused only on the reasons why you shouldn't diet. And you know what? Focusing only on the negatives is just as dreary as you might expect. So I added in a self-affirming, positive, and supportive Tip to go along with each Reason.

Use this book in ways that best support you. You can read the Reasons first and then the Tips. You can read each Reason and Tip together, try the Tip and then move on to the next one. Or you can just try the Tips. If you start to feel discouraged, mix it up a bit. You can always do the Tips that sound fun or intriguing and then go back to the other ones later. To make things easier, I've broken down these Reasons into categories—physical, emotional, mental, monetary and societal, so you can connect with those Reasons not to diet that appeal to you first.

Just keep an open mind as you decide what's best for you.

If you're someone who is new to eating without dieting, rely on the Tips to support this transition. For many of us, dieting is like an addiction. We use dieting as a way to feel in control of our lives and our bodies. As with any addiction, when you begin to break away from dieting, you may feel a sense of withdrawal—emotions come up, you feel out of control, and you're not quite sure how to go about your daily life without dieting. Use the Tips to steady yourself as you break away from dieting.

By diving into the Tips in this book, you will transform your relationship with food and your body. I see this every day with my Body Love Wellness clients. You may want to keep a journal for yourself as you try the Tips, and take note of the transformation that happens. You will be amazed at how different you feel.

A Note About Size—Or Why This Book Is So Short

I kept this book to its diminutive size because I want you to be able to keep it with you. Keep it handy for when you find yourself feeling guilty about eating something, or dealing with a diet-pushing friend, or a super skinny magazine image makes you doubt yourself. In other words, I want this book to support you rather than drag you (or your handbag) down.

Reason #1:
Let's Be Clear: Diets Don't Work

🐝🍂

D iets have such a high failure rate that they are really a gamble with a low chance of success. If you look at the fine print of most studies on diets, you will learn that diets have a 85-99% long-term (i.e., three-to-five year) failure rate. People lose some weight, only to find that it creeps back up, often surpassing their initial, pre-diet weight. Even the dieters that the studies deem "successful" often don't keep off more than a few pounds.[i] This is why you (and nearly everyone you know who has ever dieted) have gained the weight back, very often ending up at a weight that is higher than where you started. This is also why every ad for every diet, whether on television, in print or online has that darn "results not typical" disclaimer when mentioning a client who lost any amount of weight.

In other words, it wasn't your fault. The odds were greatly, and heavily, stacked against you.

So now that you know that you didn't fail at dieting because diets don't work anyway, what can you do with this information? Instead, you can use it to empower yourself. Use the knowledge that diets don't work to remind yourself that you haven't failed at anything, that you don't lack willpower or determination, and that you haven't done anything wrong.

Diets don't work, so you don't have to search for the right one or pay money to a diet guru. You can begin the process—right now—of trusting your body and knowing that, when you listen closely enough, it will tell you what it needs. (We will talk more about this process, known as *intuitive eating*, throughout the book. In the meantime, keep reading and trying some of the Tips to help you in this process of becoming re-attuned to your body.)

Tip #1:
Your Dieting History

Take a moment to write out your dieting history on the following pages. Write down what age you were when you started each diet, what the diet was, your weight when you started, your weight when you stopped, and what your beliefs about the diet were when you started and stopped. Doing this is often a huge eye opener for dieters. Consider sharing these notes with a friend to check out the similarities and differences. To give you an idea, here are two sample entries:

Age	Diet	Start Weight	End Weight	Beliefs
12-13	*Self-invented, sort of low carb*	*140 lbs*	*135 lbs (got to 130 and then came back up)*	*Thought it would make boys like me, thought I would lose more weight*
18-20	*Self-invented, sort of low fat*	*160 lbs*	*165 lbs (lost about 15 lbs then gained it back plus more.)*	*Was worried about the freshman 15 before it even happened, thought it would make college easier, tried to impress weight-focused roommate*

Age	Diet	Start Weight	End Weight	Beliefs

Age	Diet	Start Weight	End Weight	Beliefs

Now that we're clear on the fact that diets don't work, let's address some of the other negative physical, emotional, mental, monetary and societal effects of dieting, as well as some helpful ways to create change.

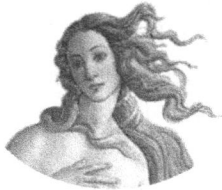

PART I:
PHYSICAL REASONS TO
STOP DIETING NOW

Reason #2:
All Diets Are Yo-Yo Diets

As we discussed in **Reason #1**, diets don't work. The vast majority of people who lose weight on a diet gain it back within three to five years or less. Since the conventional wisdom is that dieters who gain weight back should try another diet, many of them do so and repeat that cycle all over again.

In other words, if you're on a diet and have been on diets in the past, you've been yo-yo dieting.

Even diet gurus who say that they believe in the efficacy of diets believe that yo-yo dieting (also known as weight cycling) is bad for you. Weight cycling puts added stress on your heart, affects your metabolism, and depletes your immune system. In fact, more and more research shows that the weight loss/gain cycle created by dieting puts more stress on the body than just being plain, old fat.[ii]

Tip #2:
Reality Check

Take a moment and look back at your diet history from **Tip #1**. Using as much information as you have, see if you can add up all of the weight you've lost on diets and all of the weight you've regained. Does adding these amounts up give you a sense of what your body has been through as a result of dieting? Don't judge yourself for your dieting choices—you were doing the best you could with the information you had at the time. But the next time you consider starting yet another diet, ask yourself if it's worth the added stress on your body. Ask yourself if the likelihood that you'll gain the weight back, coupled with the dangers of weight cycling, are worth the teeny likelihood that you'll lose weight and keep it off permanently.

Notes - your thoughts on the dieting reality check

Reason #3:
Diets Make You Crave "Bad" Foods

✿❧

It's no accident that our culture's *Genesis* story revolves around a woman eating a forbidden food (the apple). It's human nature to want what's forbidden. So it's no wonder that dieters often crave forbidden foods even more once they are forbidden, and then hate themselves for eating those foods.

Think about it: do you have a "bad" food list? What's on this list? How do you feel when you're around foods on your bad foods list? For example, let's say you love ice cream cake but it's on your bad foods list. What happens when you're at a party and there's ice cream cake there? While you're interacting with people at the party, do you find yourself thinking about whether or not to have a piece of cake? If you don't have the cake, do you feel like you missed out later? If you do have the cake, do you feel guilty when you eat it or perhaps feel guilty later, after the party, when the good feeling of being at the party is gone? Dieting creates this type of obsessive behavior.

But here is the grim reality: you want to eat the foods on your bad foods list more than anything. You probably find yourself thinking of those foods at unexpected times. You probably see other people eating those foods and, in that moment, you hate those people for "being able" to eat those foods, or you find yourself feeling superior to them for not eating those foods. If you (or someone in your house) actually buys the foods on your bad foods list, you probably can almost hear those foods calling to you as you watch television in another room and try really, *really* hard not to think about the fact that such bad foods are so close at hand.

In other words, the more "evil" you consider the food, the more you desire it, think about it, and crave it.

Tip #3:
Savor Your "Bad" Foods

If you're a current dieter, and we were working together, I might have you make a list of your bad foods, and start asking you to eat the ones that you desire most, with the added caveat that you must savor them. I would ask you to really taste the food, going slowly, noticing flavor and texture, etc. I would ask you to do this because when you allow yourself to eat foods on your bad foods list, without guilt or shame, without self hatred, and with a focus on really tasting the food, you will find out some really interesting things. You will find out that you either (a) really like that food and want to enjoy it more or (b) never really liked it that much in the first place. If you've been dieting a long time, and you finally don't have a forbidden foods list, you may find yourself eating your forbidden foods more than you wish at first. After awhile, however, those forbidden foods lose their power over you. You no longer feel a sense of desperation around them. They no longer cause fear, or control you. Eventually, when you're at a party with ice cream cake, you're able to check in with yourself and decide whether you want the cake or not. And then you can actually spend time enjoying yourself. It's really that simple—and incredibly freeing.

Just a note—I understand that the idea of eating foods on your bad foods list is utterly frightening for many of you, and if it is, I encourage you to work with me or someone like me to support you in this process. Remember that it's always okay to ask for help and support in these areas.

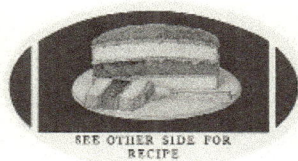

SEE OTHER SIDE FOR
RECIPE

Notes - what's on your "bad" food list?

Reason #4:
Diets Make Eating Stressful

❧

As we discussed in **Reason #3**, dieters and ex-dieters are accustomed to thinking about food in terms of "good" and "bad." You probably have a list of good foods (likely comprised of mostly very low calorie vegetables) and a longer list of bad foods (depending on your current diet, this probably includes anything with sugar or fat or carbs, and probably lots of foods that you really like).

As someone with a degree in integrative nutrition, I am, of course, an advocate for having fresh, organic, well-made food available to everyone. I believe that the more people have access to whole, non-chemicalized foods, the less prevalent certain diseases will become.

That said, the way most of us *talk* about our food may be more unhealthy than most of the food we eat. When we talk about how "bad" or "junky" or "crappy" or "unhealthy" our food is, we create an unhealthy degree of stress related to food and eating.

When you eat and think that you're eating something bad for you, it creates a stress response in the body. Your body is getting two, contradictory signals: digest this food—but don't really digest it because it's bad and poisonous! On top of these mixed signals, the stress of this conflict between what you're actually doing and what your brain thinks you should be doing creates a stress response, also known as a "fight or flight" response. When you're in fight or flight mode, the blood rushes away from the core of your body (where digestion takes place) to your limbs (where fighting and fleeing take place). As a result of stressing yourself out about what you're eating while you're eating, you become unable to fully digest your food.

Tip #4:
Have A Moment Of Food Gratitude

Whenever you eat, you want to relax your mind and body to allow for better digestion and more enjoyment of your food. Take a moment, every time you eat, to bless your food. Take a moment to thank Mother Nature, another deity, the food itself, or yourself for feeding your body and nourishing yourself so well. Make this blessing truly your own and have fun with it. You can think it to yourself or say it aloud. Getting your friends in on this will make it even more pleasurable. And if you're accustomed to already blessing your meals as part of a religious practice, pay even more attention to the words you use. Feel the gratitude for the food in your body.

Notice how this changes the way you eat, enjoy, and digest your meals.

Notes - what was the effect of blessing your food?

Reason #5:
Diet Foods Are Full Of Chemicals

Many diets support the use of non-nutritional, highly chemicalized foods like fake fats and fake sugars. These chemicalized foods negatively affect body chemistry, cause low-level under-nourishment, and often encourage overeating when the dieter gets the signal that s/he is not getting nourishment.

As an example, back when I was counting points on Weight Watchers, I developed a horrific gastrointestinal problem the likes of which I had never experienced before. I was spending the day in pain, experiencing incredible bloating and ending up in the bathroom for hours. I was frightened of what might be happening to my body, so I made an appointment with a highly recommended internist. The earliest appointment I could get was a week away.

At some point during that week, I had an inkling that I should stop eating the delicious low-fat cheese product I had been eating regularly due to its low Weight Watchers Point status. I stopped eating the cheese (I was only having a few bites of it a day) and within three days my stomach felt normal again.

I had similar experiences with diet foods—a popular ice cream bar and a diet brand name pretzel snack both caused rashes that, once I figured out the cause, disappeared within a few days. I've seen this pattern over and over again with my clients too.

Our bodies are not really designed to eat food made up mainly of chemicals. When we are able to connect with the wisdom of our bodies, we know what our bodies really crave—whole foods full of nutrients, vitamins and minerals (with the occasional piece of cake, of course!) Diet programs diminish our ability to make appropriate, real food choices.

Tip #5:
The Real Nutrition Facts

Think back to some of your recent diets. Were there any processed, chemicalized foods that you ate because they were "on your diet plan?" If you have any around, take a look at the ingredients list (not the calories/fats/carbs facts) and see if there is any *real food* in your diet food! Think about whether you would have eaten these foods if you *weren't* on a diet. And, if you're having gastrointestinal, skin or allergy issues that seemed to come from nowhere, try going off any highly processed diet foods for a few days and see if you notice a difference.

Notes - what are your thoughts on diet foods?

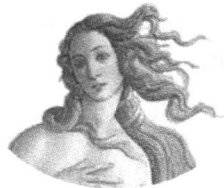

PART II:
EMOTIONAL REASONS
TO STOP DIETING NOW

Reason #6:
Diets Make You Blame Yourself
When They Don't Work
(i.e., Nearly All Of The Time)

As we discussed back in **Reason #1**, diets don't work. But when they stop working, the majority of dieters internalize the diet's failure as their own.

The last time I lost weight on a diet, I felt like I was living the dream. I had lost over 40 pounds, and, according to my Weight Watchers leader, there was nowhere to go but thinner, until I reached my goal weight. My goal weight was still higher than the "approved" weights for my height (which seemed too low for someone with my frame), but I was going to get a note from my chiropractor so that when I lost another 20 pounds or so, I'd be at my goal. I'd be roughly a size 10/12, the thinnest I had ever been.

I really thought that this time, it was going to work for me. This time, I was sure. This time, I had found the magic bullet, the pot of gold at the end of the rainbow. This time, I was going to be thin and stay thin and, as a result, have the life I was waiting to have, and love myself the way I wanted to.

I have a feeling that if you're reading this, you can relate!

As it happened, of course, I never reached my goal weight. I kept weighing and measuring food. I kept calculating points. I kept exercising to get more food points. I did everything I was supposed to do, but the number on the scale kept climbing. I couldn't raise my hand when my Weight Watchers leader asked who had lost weight this week. I clapped for everyone else but inside I felt like a failure. I felt like I had done something horribly wrong, that there was something horribly wrong with me.

Completely freaked out by my weight gain and desperate for answers, I asked my Weight Watchers leader what I was doing wrong. Her response? She asked me if I had been sick. "Cough drops," she said, "can add lots of hidden points."

I hadn't had any cough drops. I was just getting fatter. Or, re-getting fat, if you will.

At the time, I blamed myself entirely. I felt like a loser for not being able to keep off the weight. It was a horrible feeling, and I felt it mainly because I didn't know that *I wasn't the problem.*

Tip #6:
Stop Your Blame Game

The best way to stop blaming yourself for diet failures is to refer to this book often! You are constantly fed (pun intended!) a lie that diet failure is your fault. But it's not. You're not the problem. There is nothing wrong with your body. There is nothing wrong with your willpower. Nearly everyone who diets gains it all back. The sooner you can stop blaming yourself for gaining back weight, the better you can feel, right now.

Notes - how have you blamed yourself for diet failures?

Reason #7:
Diets Lower Your Self Esteem

❧

D ieters' self esteem is often tied to their weight—they feel good about themselves when they're losing weight and bad about themselves when they're gaining weight.

You know the feeling. You've been dieting. You got on the scale at home or at a meeting and you've lost a pound or two or five. You walk away from the scale, get dressed, and walk outside. You feel fantastic. The sun is a little brighter. The breeze is a little balmier. Everyone on the street is checking out your fine, fine self.

If you know that feeling, you probably also know the opposite feeling. You got on the scale at home or at a meeting and you've gained a half of a pound, or two or five. You walk outside and the sky is gray and threatening rain. A cold wind makes your bad hair day even worse. No one on the street looks at you, except to scowl.

Other than weather conditions, what really makes the difference between these two scenarios? Here's a hint: it has nothing to do with the number on the scale.

Too often we let the scale control us. We gain weight and feel terrible, worthless, unattractive, and disliked. We lose weight and suddenly feel the opposite of those things. But this pattern is not innate—it is a pattern that is deeply reinforced by dieting. A 2004 study found that chronic dieters have lowered body satisfaction and appearance evaluation than non-dieters, and those two factors create a breeding ground for low self esteem.[iv]

Golda Poretsky, H.H.C.

Tip #7:
The Mirror Check

Allowing the scale to determine how we feel about ourselves is actually a choice. The way to reverse this choice is to make a new one. Choose to know that your value is independent of how much you weigh. Your value is intrinsic and unchanging. Stop looking to the scale for an indicator of how you should feel. Decide, every day, that you are worthwhile, valuable and beautiful. Every time you pass a mirror, say aloud or think, "I am beautiful." Let this message of acknowledgement drown out the negative messages that you're more accustomed to thinking and saying. See how that affects your day.

Notes - on the mirror check. What are the effects after 1 day, 1 week, and 1 month of using this technique?

23

Stop Dieting Now: 25 Reasons to Stop, 25 Ways to Heal

Notes - on the mirror check. What are the effects after 1 day, 1 week, and 1 month of using this technique?

24

Reason #8:
Diets Make You Hate Your Body

❧

Dieters tend to see their bodies as wrong and problematic when they're not seeing the "results" they want. This causes intense body hatred that becomes more and more ingrained over time.

Contrary to what diets teach you, you are not at odds with your body. Your body is *you*. Your mind and body are connected and inextricable. When you tell yourself that your body is bad or wrong or awful, when you say you hate your thighs, when you say you hate your belly, the message you send to yourself is, "I hate myself."

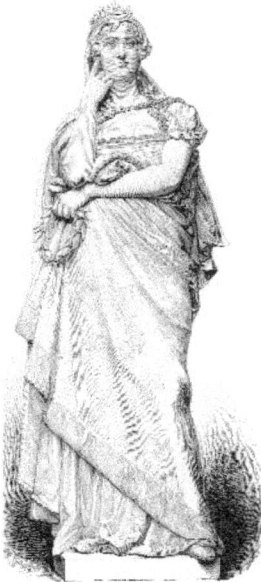

Your body is not your problem. Your body is not something to be controlled, disparaged or hated. Your body is the physical manifestation of who you are in the world. When I work with clients on shifting their relationship with their body to one of love, they immediately make better food choices and better life choices, and they start to have more fun. Their self-love is no longer tied to a number on the scale. Their self-love becomes a fact of their lives. In essence, they find the happiness that they had hoped to find from dieting. I desire this transformation for you too.

Tip #8:
Body Lovin' Self Care

Do something every day that is loving toward your body and gives you the opportunity to enjoy the sensations of your body. This could mean anything from getting a massage, to getting a hug from a loved one, to spending a little extra time applying body lotion and enjoying the sensation. Many of these things are free and take almost no time to do, but you may find yourself feeling the benefits all day long. The key is to focus in on how your body actually feels, not on how your mind thinks it should feel.

Notes - what did you try and what was it like?

Reason #9:
Diets Teach You Not To Trust Yourself And Reward You For Not Thinking For Yourself

❧

The way we relate to food and our bodies colors other aspects of our lives. If you're accustomed to dieting, you're accustomed to feeling as though you need a system of outside rules to control your life. This is particularly dangerous considering that at any given time, 115 million Americans are on a diet, the majority of whom are women[iv]. What does this mean for women when we're constantly being told that we can't be trusted to perform the basic bodily function of feeding ourselves properly?

The diet system reinforces low self esteem in dieters by making them feel like they have no "willpower" when they have diet lapses. In actuality, diets encourage people to ignore their internal will in exchange for the perceived will of the diet industry.

Dieting gives dieters the message that they cannot trust their internal sense of what nourishes them. This distrust of internal signals affects other aspects of a dieter's life, where they seek external approval and control of their non-food related actions.

Tip #9:
Actively Listening To Yourself

The way to move out of this type of thinking is to begin to trust yourself and your intuition. Start listening to your inner voice, and accept what it tells you. Act upon your inner voice. For example, if your inner voice tells you to take a different route to work or wear a different outfit than you had planned, follow it and see where it takes you. Eventually, your inner voice will speak up in relation to food choices too. With practice, you'll find your inner voice becoming louder and clearer in every facet of your life. Hearing this inner voice will help you to move out of a dieting mentality and support you in becoming an intuitive eater.

If you feel like your inner voice is too quiet to hear, just guess at what she would say and act upon that guess. You will be right more than you expect. In time and with practice, you will hear your inner voice loudly and clearly.

Notes - what is your inner voice saying and what is it like to act upon it?

Notes - what is your inner voice saying and what is it like to act upon it?

Reason #10:
Diets Make You Put Off
The Good Things You Can Have
Right Now

🍀

Do you find yourself saying, "When I lose 5/10/20/50/100 pounds, then I will finally _____? Fill in the blank for yourself. Will you finally be happy, date more, get married, get a new job, buy new clothes, or just really start living?

Dieters often reinforce their dieting behaviors by promising to do positive things for themselves once they lose a certain amount of weight. And yet, it's human nature to want things *now*. Have you ever promised yourself a certain thing once you've gotten down to a certain weight, but never reached that weight? Have you ever promised to give yourself something when you've gotten to a certain weight, only to find that once you've reached that weight, you don't even want it anymore?

Happiness is not a destination, nor is it a dress size. You have the right to life, liberty and the pursuit (and attainment) of happiness right here and now. What are you going to do with it, darling?

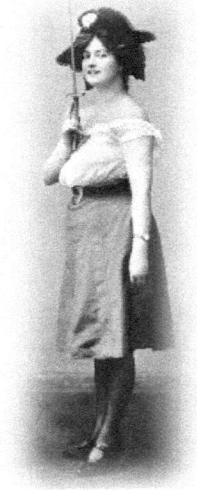

Tip #10:
Fulfill Your Desires

Take a moment to make a list of things you've been waiting to do once you lose weight. List everything you can think of—big or small. Once you have the list, systematically start fulfilling your own desires right now. Buy a new dress that fits you in the size you're at right now. Learn to SCUBA dive. Join a dating site. Start looking for your dream job. Give yourself whatever you've been putting off and telling yourself you can only have when you reach a certain weight. Enjoy those things right now. Allow yourself happiness right now. It is your birthright.

Notes - what am I "weighting" for?

Notes - what am I "weighting" for?

Golda Poretsky, H.H.C.

Reason #11:
Diets Can Be A Band-Aid
When You Really Need Stitches

🌺🍃

For some people, diets are like band-aids on deep wounds. For people who really overeat and who eat unconsciously, eating is a way to numb their feelings and go unconscious from hurtful feelings.

For example, if you find yourself binge eating somewhat regularly (i.e., eating to a point that is way past your comfort zone), your issue is not really about portion size. If you were able to slow down, you would know that your portions are bigger than what your body really wants or needs. Instead, something is happening that makes you eat more than you actually want to, because you are overriding that voice inside that tells you you're done eating.

In other words, you are likely overeating due to some form of emotional stress, not because you have no sense of appropriate portion size. If your portions feel out of control, measuring them is not the solution. It's like putting a band-aid on a deep knife wound. The wound may appear temporarily better, the bleeding may appear to have stopped, but soon enough you'll notice that this wound needs much more attention. Additionally, just putting a band-aid on it may have led to more problems than addressing the problem right away. By putting a band-aid on it, you're just attending to a minor symptom of a more dangerous problem.

Overeating from emotional stress is a complex coping mechanism. At some point in your life, you found that it was not acceptable to inhabit and/or reveal your emotional reality, and found solace in food. This is an extremely common coping mechanism, one that should be handled thoroughly and compassionately by an appropriate counselor, not by a dietary regulation of portion control. Overcoming emotional overeating often requires that the overeater get more in touch with their emotions and start expressing them. In other words, they need to control themselves *less*, not more. Portion control is just another form of control.

Tip #11:
Break Time!

If you find yourself going unconscious when you eat (for example, not noticing how much you're eating, not tasting your food, knowing that you're unhappy but not wanting to address it and eating instead) know that you can stop. As soon as you notice that you're eating unconsciously, take a moment to think "I can stop," and stop. Stop eating. Take a breath. Take another breath. Then ask yourself this question, "Am I hungry for food or something else?" Pay attention to the answer. If the answer is "I'm hungry for food," then eat, and enjoy and savor your food. If the answer is "something else," ask yourself what that is, and try to give it to yourself. For example, if you're feeling lonely, stop to call a friend or write an email. If you're feeling angry, see if there is a safe way to voice your concerns, or at least get your feelings out into a journal. The more adept you become at asking this question, the more you will find answers. And remember, no matter what the answer, treat yourself with love and don't judge yourself, even if the answer is, "Leave me alone, I just want to eat unconsciously for a while!" The more you judge yourself harshly, the more you will want to address the pain of this judgment with eating unconsciously.

Notes - what have you noticed about checking in with your hunger?

Reason #12:
Diets Makes Food About Reward
And Punishment

🍂

Dieters are masters of unintentional sado-masochism. Have you ever punished yourself with too little food? Too much food? Have you ever rewarded yourself with something because you've been so good—or not let yourself enjoy food because you've been so bad?

Rather than being about nourishment, food often becomes about reward and punishment for dieters. Dieting tells us that there are "good" and "bad" foods. So when we eat good foods and adhere to our diet, we are good, right, moral, and possibly deserving of a treat. When we eat bad foods, we are bad, evil, immoral, embarrassing, shameful, and therefore not deserving of a treat— perhaps not even deserving of good treatment.

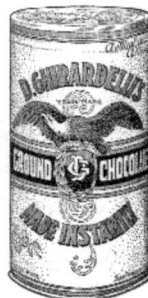

Imagine, instead, a world where food is neutral. In this world, food is about what your body needs and desires right now. In this world, you could eat delicious, healthy, whole foods all week, and find at the end of the week that you don't really want a treat. In this world, you could have a stressful week, eat some junk food, find yourself at a party, and still enjoy a piece of cake, because *you want it*. It's that simple. You're not bad when you eat "badly" or good when you eat healthfully. You don't need to be punished or given treats.

In other words, you are an adult. As an adult, you are capable of paying attention to your needs and eating in accordance with them. You don't need to be encouraged to eat well or punished for poor eating. You are entitled to maintain a positive sense of self no matter your actions.

And as an adult, you also understand that *punishment doesn't work*. Punishment doesn't create long term "good behavior". Punishment makes you feel bad, ashamed, and hurt. And if you're like most people, when you feel that way, you find solace from that pain—to some extent—in food.

Tip #12:
The Neutrality Pact

Stop being intentionally hurtful to yourself by using food as rewards or punishments. When you start treating food in this way, notice your thoughts and say (in your head or aloud) "Cancel!" Then replace the thought with a positive one, like "I always treat my body with love." Find a way to move toward self-love no matter where your actions take you. The results will be much more healing than a diet ever could be.

Notes - on how you use food to reward and/or punish yourself

Notes - on how you use food to reward and/or punish yourself

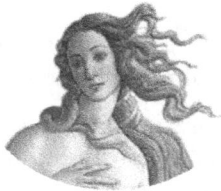

PART III:
MENTAL REASONS TO
STOP DIETING NOW

Reason #13:
Diets Create Anorectic Thinking

Some of the hallmark symptoms of anorexia are an obsession with losing weight, a deep fear of being fat or becoming more fat, distorted body image, and voluntarily ignoring one's own hunger signals.

Do these symptoms sound familiar to you? I know firsthand that I experienced them almost all the time as a dieter.

Of course, with anorexia, these symptoms are taken to an extreme. However, if you've ever been on a diet, you've probably experienced one or more of these symptoms yourself, and dieting encourages these symptoms.

For many people, dieting is like a "gateway drug" into anorexia and bulimia. While dieting, they first learn to obsess about how much they weigh, what they eat, and how much they eat.

They are taught to override their hunger and substitute their desires with the requirements of the diet.

In other words, even if dieting doesn't lead to full blown anorexia, it does lead to anorectic type thinking and obsessing about food and weight. As you can imagine, this is not the type of "healthy behavior" that most people think dieting creates!

Tip #13:
Acknowledge Your Thoughts

Spend some time over the course of a day or a few days writing down your thoughts and feelings about food and eating. Do you find yourself feeling guilty for eating? Do you find yourself judging yourself or someone else for what they eat? Then spend some time over the course of a day or a few days noticing and writing down your thoughts about your body. Do you think negative thoughts about your body or parts of your body? Do you find yourself engaging in jealous or judgmental thoughts about other people's bodies? Bringing awareness to these thoughts is the first step in releasing them and choosing thoughts that feel better to you. You may be surprised at how many negative thoughts about your body and food go through your mind each day or each hour.

Notes - when you pay attention, what recurring thoughts do you have about <u>food</u>?

Notes - when you pay attention, what recurring thoughts do you have about your <u>body</u>?

Golda Poretsky, H.H.C.

Reason #14:
Diet Programs Make You Feel Like You Don't Know How To Eat When You're Not On A Diet

❧

You probably know this feeling. You've decided to get off your most recent diet completely, because it stopped working for you, and now you're more nervous around food than you ever were before.

That's because each diet contains a system of rules, some of which often conflict completely. For example, if you do a low carbohydrate diet, you've learned to avoid bread, pasta, certain vegetables, etc. Let's say that diet stops working. You go off the diet for a while (feeling unsteady around food and possibly binging to compensate for what you've been missing) and then you run into a friend who tells you that the low carbohydrate route didn't work for her, but now she's on Weight Watchers and she's lost fifty pounds. So you decide to sign up for Weight Watchers and suddenly carbohydrates are okay again, but you have to lower your fat intake. This works at first (until it *doesn't*) and you go off the diet or begin the search for another one. All of this can happen over a period of months, years, or decades.

You may have tried lots of diets or gotten conflicting advice from friends, doctors, or nutritionists. So what happens to you when you decide to go off a diet? You feel guilty for "failing" at something that has failed you. You have conflicting rules in your head about what you should eat and what you shouldn't eat. And in the end, food stresses you out, so that you may find yourself ignoring it altogether (starving) or going numb while eating (binging). These problems are actually caused, to a great extent, by dieting, but often dieters only find solace from these effects by going on yet another diet and continuing the cycle.

Tip #14:
Rules Are Made To Be Broken

Take a moment to write out all of the diet rules that you still hear in your mind. Do you still follow some of them even if you're off the diet? Do some of them conflict and yet you still try to follow them? Do some of them seem crazy? Having an awareness of the diet rules that still haunt your choices will help you to release them and make choices based on what your body desires. Like in **Tip #12** and **Tip #15**, when these old diet rules come up for you, think "Cancel" and then listen in for what your body really desires.

Notes - what are your lingering diet rules?

Reason #15:
Diets Put The Focus On Weight As The Sole Indicator Of Health

If you pick up a newspaper, watch television or just pass a billboard occasionally, then you've taken in lots of information about the "obesity epidemic" and the horrendous things that some scientists have linked to being fat: joint problems, diabetes, heart disease, and in some instances, even cancer.

In reality, however, there are many, many studies (especially ones that are not paid for by the diet industry) that find that there isn't a correlation between these illnesses and fatness. Even more intriguing, there is little evidence to show that losing weight lessens the risks or symptoms of any of these diseases for any length of time.

So to counter all the bad information you've received throughout your life, here is some food for thought on a number of diseases that, until now, you've been told to live in fear of because of your weight.

Cardiovascular Disease: Reviews of major studies on hypertension show no link between weight loss and a reduction in hypertension. Additionally, studies show that yo-yo dieting causes more cardiovascular problems than just being fat. In fact, a recent study found that being overweight or obese may protect individuals from cardiac death.

Diabetes: Those involved in the "War On Fat" often claim that diabetes is on the rise. Other researchers, however, say that it is not on the rise, but that the definition has changed (i.e., the fasting blood sugar level required to determine type II diabetes has been lowered) and that diabetes used to be highly under-diagnosed.[vi]

Cancer: Having a higher weight may actually protect you from some types of cancer. Fat people who eat healthfully and exercise may be better off than thin people who eat healthfully and exercise, with respect to certain cancers.[vii]

Mortality Overall: People with a BMI in the "overweight" category actually live the longest—even longer than people in the "normal weight" category. People in the "underweight category" (which includes many models and actresses) actually have the shortest lifespan—even shorter than people in the "morbidly obese" category.[viii]

Your fat also may be *protecting* you from certain diseases. Fat people have lower rates of osteoporosis, emphysema, chronic obstructive pulmonary disease, hip fracture, tuberculosis, anemia, peptic ulcer and chronic bronchitis.[ix]

The medical community often tells fat people that losing weight is the key to health. But as more and more studies show, trying to make a fat person thin can lead to more health problems than just being fat. There is also little evidence to suggest that the health benefits that thin people (arguably) enjoy are not actually bestowed upon fat people for those periods when they have dieted down to a "thin" weight.

How can you be empowered by this in-formation? By reframing what it means to be healthy. You can finally let go of thinness as a measure of your health. You can eat good food because it feels good, not because it will make you thin. You can move your body because if feels good and not because it will make you thin. You can make the changes that you want to make because you will feel better and healthier, and you don't have to drop those things if they don't lead to weight loss.

Tip #15:
Recognize Your Health

The next time you find yourself connecting fat with ill health and disease, say "Cancel!" to yourself and replace the thought with something positive, like:

"Every cell of my body is filled with health and healing."

"My body is strong, powerful, and healthy."

"I love that I am so healthy."

Create your own affirmations by reframing any recurring negative thoughts (look back at the thoughts you wrote down in **Tip #13** for inspiration) and turning them into positives. For example, if your negative thought is, "my weight is bad for my heart," turn it around to say, "my heart is healthy and vital." Remember to keep your affirmations in the present tense too. You want to think, "my heart is healthy and vital" instead of "my heart will be healthy and vital." Try it and see how much better you feel!

Notes - what are your new body positive affirmations?

Reason #16:
Diets Don't Let You Think About Anything Other Than Diets

❧

Diets cause dieters (who are often women) to build their lives around food rather than other things that may really matter to them (relationships, careers, social issues).

When you're on a diet, how much time do you spend thinking and talking about dieting? Do you talk to you friends about points, calories, carbs and fat grams? Do you find yourself working out complicated math equations in your head just to decide what to eat?

Now, imagine a world where you talked to your friends about their lives, their dreams, and their desires. Take a moment to think about how much time per day you think about dieting, how much time you take to weigh or measure your food, how much time you spend thinking about fat grams, carbs, calories, points, etc. Add that to how much time you spend worrying about what you ate or what you will eat and whether you've gone off your diet or not. How much time per day is that? If you're like most dieters, you probably spend at least an hour a day, if not more, thinking about, talking about and feeling guilty about your diet.

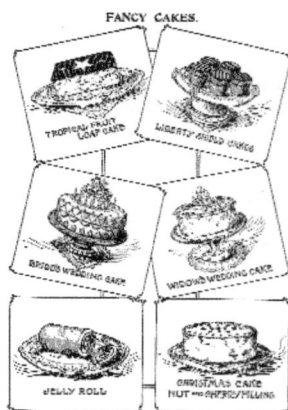

FANCY CAKES.

Tip #16:
Envision Your Diet-Free Life

If you're a dieter, imagine what you could do with all the time that is taken up by dieting. You might use it to meditate, to get your work done more efficiently, to spend time enjoying your friends, or to think about causes and concerns that are really meaningful. In other words, imagine spending that time envisioning and creating a better life for yourself—one that doesn't revolve around diets. Keep envisioning your world without dieting until your reality and your vision become one.

Notes - what would your diet-free life look like?

Reason #17:
Diets Encourage "Lottery Thinking"

Most dieters know that diets haven't really worked for them or for most of the people they know, yet they think that this new diet is going to make them thin, and they'll finally be in that tiny successful group.

If you're a chronic dieter, think back to the last diet you started. I'll bet you found yourself thinking something like, "I know that my last diet didn't work, but I'm sure this new one will!" Most chronic dieters, when they start a new diet, find themselves in that honeymoon period where they discredit their old diets and believe that they've finally found the answer in this new diet. Now think back to the diet before your current diet—do you remember thinking that that diet was the answer and that the diet before *that* was hopelessly flawed?

In other words, you always think your current diet is definitely going to work for you, until it stops working. This lottery thinking is a dangerous paradigm for dieters—it causes them to continually make the same mistake (i.e., dieting) by disregarding the reality of their prior experiences.

Tip #17:
Thought Pattern Review

You can avoid "lottery thinking" by thinking about your dieting history (and if you've already done **Tip #1**, take another look at it). Think about your thought processes when starting the diet, during the honeymoon phase, during the plateau or regaining phases, and after. What patterns do you notice? The next time you consider starting a new diet, think about your dieting history (and the other 24 Reasons in this book) and assess, with honesty, whether you really want to start another diet.

Notes - what kind of "lottery thinking" have you experienced with dieting?

Reason #18:
Diets Evoke Scarcity Thinking

❧

If you're a dieter (or if you used to be a dieter) think about how it feels, emotionally, to be on a diet. When you're on a diet, do you constantly feel like you can't have what you want? Do you get so focused on losing weight that you assume that you have to be a certain weight before you can have something?

Diets work on a scarcity principle. Diets make dieters focus on lack, tell them they can only have "this much and no more" and that to want more is a bad thing. Because dieting is so all-encompassing, this scarcity principle often filters into other aspects of dieters' lives. They begin to see lack and scarcity in their relationships, in their jobs, and in the world.

Focusing on abundance, on possibilities, on there being enough for everyone, is a very powerful framework for feeling good about one's life. I often find that when my clients start focusing on what is good about their lives, that sense of happiness—and indeed, those good things themselves—continue to grow. Alternatively, when they focus on what is wrong in their lives, and on what they need but can't have, their worldview and happiness continue to shrink. Dieting perpetuates this type of negative thinking, which is incredibly damaging to dieters' happiness.

Tip #18:
Creating Gratitude

Spend some time making a list of things you're thankful for having, rather than wish you had. You can make a general list, or a list that focuses on your body (or some other area of your life that you feel negative about, like your career or your relationship). Start each item with "I am grateful for." I like my gratitude lists to be at least ten items long. Just to make sure you get the idea, here's one of my sample lists about my body:

1. *I am grateful for my gorgeous body.*

2. *I am grateful for my strong legs.*

3. *I am grateful for my long, beautiful hair.*

4. *I am grateful for my big, sturdy feet.*

5. *I am grateful for my soft skin.*

6. *I am grateful for the way the cut on my finger is healing.*

7. *I am grateful my curvaceous hips.*

8. *I am grateful for my kissable lips.*

9. *I am grateful for my bodacious booty.*

10. *I am grateful for the way my heart pumps blood so beautifully.*

As you can see, I did a few things in my list. I focused on and reaffirmed my beauty and I turned around anything that I might find to be negative. For example, when I was a kid, I hated my big feet (my shoe size was the same as my age until I was 11!). But in my gratitude list, I shifted that toward a feeling of gratitude. Try this out. It will definitely change your mood, make you feel more positive, and allow you to focus on the abundance of all you have!

One final note—if the word "gratitude" doesn't turn you on, substitute it with "appreciation." Start each item in your list with "I appreciate _____" instead.

Notes - what are you grateful for?

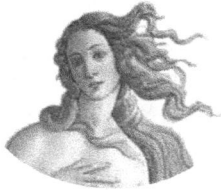

PART IV:
ECONOMIC REASONS TO
STOP DIETING NOW

Reason #19:
The Diet Industry Needs You To Fail

The diet industry has a deep interest in the failure of dieters—if everyone got skinny, they'd go out of business.

Think about how many diet programs are out there. They all say that they have the answer. They all say that even though you've tried other diet programs, their program is the one that really works. If they were all right, wouldn't everyone be thin by now? If only one were right, wouldn't all the other ones go out of business?

And in case you're wondering where the myth that dieting works comes from—the diet industry (which includes the diet drug and weight loss surgery industry) has paid for and supported pretty much all of the "research" that proves dieting works.[x]

Tip #19:
Media Studies

Spend a little time paying attention to diet company ads in newspapers and magazines, and on television and the Internet. Do they all promise the same thing? Do you notice anything interesting in the "fine print" of these ads? One of my favorite diet advertising disclaimers is "results not typical." After reading **Reason #1**, you know why!

Allow yourself to be empowered by this knowledge. You don't have to spend money on their products or plans any more, and you don't have to feel guilty or desperate when you don't spend the money. How liberating!

Notes - what do you notice about diet ads?

Reason #20:
Diets Are A Waste Of Your Money

❦

The diet industry is a sixty-billion-dollar-a-year industry in the United States alone![xi] Sixty billion dollars a year! That's over two hundred dollars for every person over eighteen years old! That number does not even include the money that people spend on weight loss surgeries, which is growing every year.[xii]

Most diet programs are expensive. I cringe when I think about the money that I and my friends and family have spent over the years on Weight Watchers, diet books, special shakes and diet pills!

I know that many of the people that push this weight loss stuff (especially those earnest "weight loss coaches") are well-meaning, but they're still peddling a bunch of crap. Even if their program caused them to lose weight, or helped a couple of their clients to lose weight, it probably won't help *you* lose weight and keep it off. So if you try their program out and you don't lose weight or gain back what you do lose, and they shift the blame back to you and tell you that you must be doing something wrong, please don't say I didn't warn you.

Tip #20:
Show Me The Money

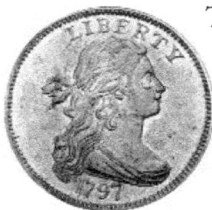

Think about the money you've spent on diet programs over the years. Have you spent hundreds, thousands, or tens of thousands on weight loss products? Imagine what that money might have meant to you at the time and what it would mean to you now. What would you do with that money if you had it all back?

Hopefully, after reading this book, you wouldn't spend it on another diet program!

Notes - what might you have done with the money you've spent on diets?

Reason #21:
Diet Programs Are Constantly Trying To Convince You That They're Not Diets, Because You Know That They Really Don't Work Anyway

Have you ever noticed how dieting companies are always trying to convince you that they're not promoting a diet? From Weight Watchers to Jenny Craig to your local diet guru, they're all trying to convince you that their program is not a diet but a lifestyle choice, a plan for living, a healthy living program, etc.

After reading the other **Reasons** in this book, you know why the diet companies do this! Because diets don't work!

Tip #21:
Put 'Em On The Spot

To help you avoid this dieting trap, ask your-self (or the diet pusher) these questions:

- Are you going to tell me what to eat in any way?

- Do I need to count something (calories, fat grams, carbs, points, starches, proteins, etc.)?

- Do I have to track my weight?

- Do I have to eat a non-food item as part of the program (bars, shakes, drugs, supplements)?

- Is the goal of this program weight loss?

If they answer "yes" to any of these questions (or try to avoid the questions all together) then it's a diet. In which case, refer to the other 24 **Reasons** in this book before you sign up.

Notes - Interview with the Vampire (er,...Diet Guru)

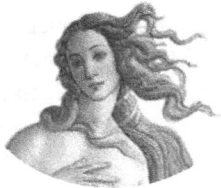

PART V:
SOCIETAL REASONS TO
STOP DIETING NOW

Reason #22:
Diets Put A Premium On
"Staying Small"

In Western culture, we take the desirability of thinness as a given, particularly for women.

If we look at American history over the last forty or so years, we find that the ultra thin ideal for women started right around the time that the women's movement infiltrated mainstream culture. In other words, as women began to occupy the male-dominated business space more and more, the societal expectation was that women themselves should take up less space.

The value and desirability of thinness is not a given. It is a problematic cultural norm that we view as normal only because it permeates our society. Consider this study: in 2002, scientists reported that the introduction of television in Fiji completely changed women's views of their bodies. Prior to the introduction of television, most Fijian women were satisfied with the way they looked no matter what their sizes. Less than a year after television became available, at least 77% of women reported dissatisfaction with their bodies and a desire to lose weight. In fact, there were no reported cases of anorexia or bulimia in Fiji until television was introduced!

By becoming aware of this cultural norm of thinness and physical smallness, you can counteract it. There is nothing wrong with taking up space, whether you're a woman or a man. Make the decision to enjoy the way you take up space. There is no need to apologize for it or make yourself smaller than you are!

Tip #22:
The Deliciously Desirable Game

This **Tip** is one of my personal favorites. The next time you find yourself in a situation where you're feeling negative about your body size, decide that your body (or the part of your body that you're particularly stressed out about) is the sexiest in the world. Whether it's your big ole butt that's bothering your or your body in general, decide that it is super sexy. Imagine that everywhere you go, people are kicking themselves wondering how you got that big, gorgeous butt or that scintillating round figure. Imagine that famous actresses are desperate to find out your secret. Then, act accordingly. You will not believe how this can shift your mood from one of despair to delight.

Notes - what did it feel like to play the "Deliciously Desirable" game?

Reason #23:
The Myth That Diets Work
Makes Size Discrimination Acceptable

❧

A 2008 study found that there was a 50 percent increase in size discrimination from 1996 to 2006 and that size discrimination is as common as racial discrimination.[xiv] From what I see, the myth that dieting works helps to support this discrimination.

Most people out there haven't read this book or other books on the problems with dieting. Consequently, most people think that dieting works.

Now, if you're someone who assumes dieting works, what do you then assume about fat people? You probably assume that they're lazy and eat loads of junk food and never exercise. You probably assume that fat people have never dieted or done anything about their "weight problem."

In other words, if you think dieting works, then you can associate lots of negative things with fat people. If dieting works, then fat people are making a choice to live outside of cultural norms and therefore, in some people's minds, they are worthy of discrimination. It's a similar mindset to some people's approach to homosexuality; i.e., we don't need to extend marriage rights to gay people because they could just decide not to be gay.

As most gay people will tell you, being gay is not usually a choice. Similarly, as most fat people will tell you, being fat is not usually a choice. It's just a reality. And the more that people understand this, and the more people understand that dieting doesn't work, the more hope there is to stem discrimination against fat people.

Tip #23: Fight For Your Rights

Check out the National Association To Advance Fat Acceptance (NAAFA) web site (www.NAAFA.org) for more information on their anti-discrimination efforts. Take part in local efforts to get anti-discrimination legislation on the books in your state. Feel good about doing your part to end size discrimination!

Notes - how would you like to fight for your rights?

Reason #24:
Diets Don't Account For Size Diversity

❧

D iets assume that all fat people eat too much. They don't account for the fact that people naturally come in a variety of shapes and sizes.

You know you have skinny friends who eat way more than you do. You probably also have fat friends who eat way less than you do. I'm sure you can think of many thin people who eat a lot, fat people who don't eat a lot, and people who fall somewhere in between.

Most diet gurus assume that fat people—even if they don't eat a lot when they're in public—go home and binge eat when nobody's looking. And it's true that some fat people do that, but not all fat people. It's also true that some thin people do that.

So in other words, going on a restrictive diet to lose weight doesn't really make sense for all fat people, because plenty of fat people don't overeat (and even if they do, restrictive diets are not the answer). Some fat people are just fat because that's how they're made, or because of medicine they take, or because they spent years on diets that hurt their metabolism. By the same token, some thin people are thin despite the fact that they overeat. Thin people are often thin because that's how they're made, or because of medication, or because they never messed up their metabolism with dieting.

Just as there are tall people and short people and medium height people, there are thin people and fat people and medium weight people. And just as we wouldn't think that a tall person should try to get shorter, or must be morally deficient because they got so tall, or must have no willpower because they got so tall, we shouldn't think these things of fat people. The more we allow for and celebrate size diversity, the more we allow people to accept who they are.

Tip 24:
Seeing The Beauty

Spend some time appreciating and noticing the beauty in different sorts of bodies. Start searching for beauty and you will begin to see it everywhere. You might find adorableness in a petite wrist and a plump forearm. You might find a strikingly gorgeous quality about one person's rounded fat rolls and another's rounded six pack abs. In other words, start looking for the gorgeousness that is inherent in each person—whether big or small, fat or thin—and you will begin to see it and appreciate it in yourself as well.

Notes - where did you see the beauty?

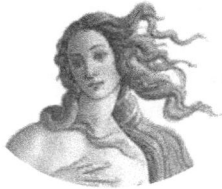

PART VI:
PLEASE STOP DIETING
NOW BECAUSE . . .

Reason #25:
Dieting Is Just A Misguided Attempt at Finding Happiness

Why do you want to be thin, or thinner? Do you think being thin or thinner will make you a success in business? Do you think it will help you find a better mate? A more attractive mate? Do you think it will make you healthier? Do you think it will make you sexier, more interesting, more fun? In other words, do you assume that on that fateful day, when you reach your goal weight and have the body you want, you will finally be truly happy?

In essence, this is why all of us have dieted. We have bought into the myth that being thin means finally being permanently happy.

The reality is, of course, that thinness does not equal happiness. Thin people still have problems, go bankrupt, get divorced, get sick, and eventually, die.

Now, you may be shaking your head as you read this. You may be thinking, "But I was happier when I was thinner!"

I can't really disagree with you, of course. You may have been happier when you were thinner. But I want you to think about that time a little more. Were you happier because you were thinner or because when you were thinner you felt better about yourself? When you were thinner, did you date more, have more fun, wear nicer clothes? And if so, could you do all of those things right now? Could you make your health and your happiness a priority without assuming that you need to lose weight to do it?

You dieted because you thought it would make you happy, but it didn't. So now let's let go of diets, once and for all, and give Plan B a shot. Are you with me?

Tip #25: Fat And Happy

Take a moment to get really clear on your desires. Write out what you want and what would make you happy, even if it doesn't seem attainable. Keep an ongoing journal of desires and write "Thank You!" next to each of them as they come true.

Being clear about what makes you happy will help you shift away from the belief that you need to be thin to have what you want, and will help you get clear as well on what you need right now. When you're clear on what you want, you can finally start to attain it, no matter what size you happen to be.

Notes - list your desires!

Notes - list your desires!

SO IF I STOP DIETING, WHAT DO I DO NOW?

The longer you've dieted, the harder it can be to get off the dieting roller coaster forever. But you can do it, and here's how.

Start With The Tips: Try each Tip in this book. Do them in order, starting with the first, or do the one that appeals to you most first. Try each one. See how you feel. See which ones resonate with you and which ones don't. Use these Tips as a guidepost away from dieting and toward a new way of life that is centered on *your* needs and desires.

Be Gentle With Yourself: Once you get clear that you don't want to diet anymore, be gentle with yourself. Start listening to what your inner voice tells you and start acting on that inner voice. Your inner voice may be quiet at first, but make a commitment to listen for it. Be gentle and patient and willing to focus on finding inward guidance.

Get Support: Shifting away from dieting and toward intuitive eating can be difficult, particularly if you don't have a community of non-dieters to support you. Luckily, the Internet and books like these are making it easier for all of us to get together.

Find an intuitive eating counselor in your area, or get in touch with me! Through my company, Body Love Wellness (www.BodyLoveWellness.com), I provide a wide range of support, from teleclasses to individual counseling. Even if you can't come to my office in NYC, I offer telephone sessions and teleclasses for clients nationally and internationally. As my gift to you, go to page 82 to retrieve your gift certificate for a free Body Love Breakthrough Session.

Finally, don't be afraid to share your newfound knowledge with your friends. Pass this book around. Give it out as a gift. In the process, you will create your own community of women and men who reject dieting and choose to eat and live intuitively. The non-dieting revolution needs you, and you and your body needs it too. Welcome!

Additional Notes

Additional Notes

Additional Notes

_____

_____

_____

_____

_____

_____

_____

_____

_____

_____

_____

_____

_____

_____

_____

_____

Additional Notes

Notes

[i] Campos, Paul. *The Obesity Myth: Why America's Obsession with Weight Is Hazardous To Your Health*. 1st. New York: Gotham Books, 2004. 28-29. Print.
Mann, Traci, A. Janet Tomiyama, Westlin Erika, Lew Ann-Marie, Samuels Barbra, and Jason Chatman. "Medicare's Search For Effective Obesity Treatments: Diets Are Not The Answer." *American Psychologist*. 62.3 (2007): 220-233. Print.

[ii] (Campos x, 32)

[iii] Gingras, Jacqui, Jasmine Fitzpatrick, and Linda McCargar. "Body Image Of Chronic Dieters: Lowered Appearance Evaluation and Body Satisfaction." *Journal Of The American Dietetic Association*. 104.10 (2004): 1589-1592. Print.

[iv] (Campos 28-29)

[v] Kang , X, LJ Shaw, SW Hayes, R Hachamovitch, A Abidov, I Cohen, JD Friedman, LE Thomson, D Polk, G Germano, and DS Berman. "Impact Of Body Mass Index On Cardiac Mortality In Patients With Known Or Suspected Coronary Artery Disease Undergoing Myocardial Perfusion Single-Photon Emission Computed Tomography." *Journal Of The American College Of Cardiology*. 47.7 (2006): 1418-26. Web. 22 Nov 2009.

[vi] (Campos 132-33)

[vii] (Campos 22-23)

[viii] Gaesser, Glenn A. *Big Fat Lies: The Truth About Your Weight And Your Health*. 2nd. Carlsbad, CA: Gurze Books, 2002. 99-102. Print.

[ix] (Campos 23-24)

[x] (Campos 14-15)

[xi] (Gaesser 102)

xii For a more in depth discussion, check out Fraser, Laura. *Losing It: False Hopes And Fat Profits.* 1st. New York: Plume, 1998. 209-32. Print.

xiii Dahl, Jonathan, Trevor Delaney and Lisa Scherzer. "10 Things the Weight-Loss Industry Won't Say." *Smart Money* n. pag. Web. 31 Mar 2010. <http://www.smartmoney.com/spending/deals/10-things-the-weight-loss-industry-wont-tell-you-13677/>.

xiv More and more people have been writing about the dangers of weight loss surgery (including the high risk of death). For a look at a recent study, see Flum, David R., Leon Salem, Jo Ann Broeckel Elrod, E. Patchen Dellinger, Allen Cheadle, and Leighton Chan. "Early Mortality Among Medicare Beneficiaries Undergoing Bariatric Surgical Procedures." *Journal Of The American Medical Association.* 294.15 (2005): 1903-1908. Print.

xv Puhl, Rebecca, T. Andreyeva and K. D. Brownell. "Perceptions of Weight Discrimination: Prevalence and Comparison to Race and Gender Discrimination in America." *International Journal of Obesity.* (2008). Print.

A Free Offer For You

Because I'm committed to you transforming your relationship with food and your body, I've decided to offer a free Body Love Breakthrough Session to you just for reading this book.

These are the amazing benefits that you can expect from your Body Love Breakthrough Session. You'll:

- ♥ Create a sense of clarity about the way you desire to feel about your body.

- ♥ Find out the essential building blocks for having the relationship with food and your body that you've dreamed of.

- ♥ Discover the #1 thing stopping you from accepting your body and healing your relationship with food.

- ♥ Identify the most powerful actions that will move you towards the relationship with food and your body that you desire.

- ♥ Complete the consultation with the excitement of knowing exactly what you need to do to feel great about your body and heal your relationship with food.

Ready to get started? Just "clip" the coupon below by going to http://www.bodylovewellness.com/stopdietingnow-gift/ and signing up for your free session.

You Are Entitled to
(and Deserve!)
A FREE Body Love Breakthrough Session

To claim yours, go to
http://www.bodylovewellness.com/stopdietingnow-gift

ABOUT THE AUTHOR

After spending almost her entire life dieting, Golda decided in 2007 to stop dieting and start listening to her body. In 2008, she founded Body Love Wellness (www.bodylovewellness.com), incorporating her knowledge of holistic health with her belief that health and body love and acceptance are possible at every size. She now counsels women and men on how to get off the dieting roller coaster, give their bodies what they really crave, and love their bodies and themselves.

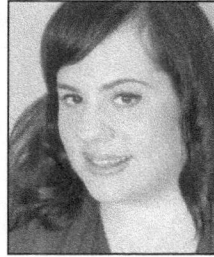

In addition to her work counseling women and men throughout the country, Golda teaches workshops and teleclasses on healthy eating without dieting, intuitive eating, and radical body love. She is also a featured weekly columnist on the web site More of Me to Love (www.moreofmetolove.com). You can also find her weekly podcast on iTunes.

Golda's counseling and activism work have been featured on CBS' "The Early Show," ABC's "Nightline," *Time Out New York* and The Huffington Post.

Golda has a degree in health counseling and integrative nutrition from the Institute for Integrative Nutrition, as well as B.A. in history from New York University and a J.D. from New York University School of Law.

Golda lives and works shakes what her Momma gave her in New York City.

www.ingramcontent.com/pod-product-compliance
Lightning Source LLC
Chambersburg PA
CBHW021342290326
41933CB00037B/541